**DO NOT REMOVE
CARDS FROM POCKET**

1/94

Everything You Need To Know About

DIET FADS

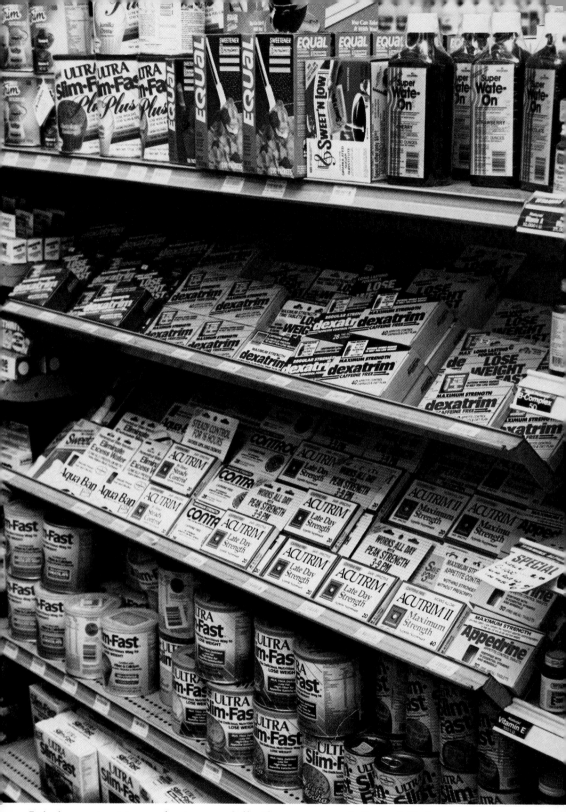

It is important to evaluate carefully the many varieties of diet products that are available.

Everything You Need To Know About

DIET FADS

Karen Bornemann Spies

THE ROSEN PUBLISHING GROUP, INC.
NEW YORK

Published in 1993 by The Rosen Publishing Group, Inc.
29 East 21st Street, New York, NY 10010

First Edition
Copyright © 1993 by The Rosen Publishing Group, Inc.

Manufactured in the United States of America.

Library of Congress Cataloging-in-Publication Data

Spies, Karen Bornemann.
    Everything you need to know about diet fads / Karen
Bornemann Spies — 1st ed.
    (The Need to know library)
    Includes bibliographical references and index.
    ISBN 0-8239-1533-6
    Summary: Discusses weight control, causes of overeating, the
dangers of diet fads, and proper nutrition.
    1. Reducing diets—Juvenile literature. 2. Teenagers—
Nutrition—Juvenile literature. [1. Weight control. 2. Nutrition.
3. Diet.] I. Title.
RM222.2.S676   1993
613.2'5—dc20   93-3415
                                                            CIP
                                                            AC

Contents

Introduction

Are you satisfied with your present weight? Many young people think that they have to be thin in order to be attractive. Fashion magazines and television sitcoms show very slim models and actresses. Good things in life are pictured as happening only to thin people. Ads, movies, and TV show fat people as lazy or lacking self-control.

These ideas, as well as pressure from other teens, make many kids feel that they *must* be thin. If not, they fear they will not be popular. In a recent study, nearly nine out of ten 17-year-old girls said that they were on a diet. But less than one in five was really overweight.

Unfortunately, at the same time that extreme thinness has become so desirable, the average teen has become less active physically. Many teens spend much more time watching television. Many drive or ride in a car rather than walk or bike to wherever they go. Many teens do not participate in any regular exercise program or team sport.

When you don't burn calories with exercise, the only way to reduce weight is to eat less. As a result, hundreds of articles and books have been written about dieting.

Diets based on good nutrition can be very helpful. But many are *crash* or *fad diets,* which are not only unhealthy, but can be dangerous. Fad diets focus on losing a lot of weight in a short time. They often recommend foods from a limited number of food groups. Some diets allow eating only one kind of food. A healthy balance of grains, fruits, and vegetables is not allowed. A healthy variety of foods eaten in smaller portions for weight control is not suggested. These diets can injure your health and cause serious problems.

If you are reading this book, chances are:

- you are curious about diets and dieting.
- you have questions about your weight.
- you have a friend with a weight problem.
- you want help planning your diet.

This book will provide you with some important information. You will learn ways to feel good about yourself and your body. You will learn how to eat when you're hungry—and only when you're hungry. Most important, you will learn how to develop habits that will help you keep your weight under control for the rest of your life.

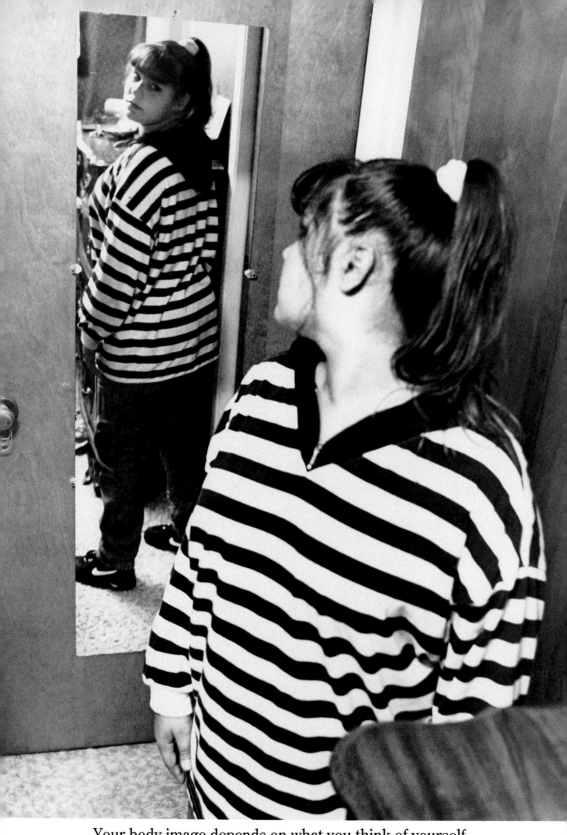

Your body image depends on what you think of yourself.

Chapter 1

How Much Should I Weigh?

F *or as long as Kristy could remember, she had been the fattest girl in her class. Whenever a new diet came out, Kristy was one of the first to try it. One month she ate nothing but bananas. The next month she tried eating grapefruit and drinking water. She would lose a few pounds, but then she'd get so hungry that she'd eat everything in sight. Kristy wondered if she'd ever be able to lose weight and keep it off. She thought that was the only way anyone would ever want to be her friend.*

Terry had always wanted to be popular. He didn't want to be known only as a "brain." But he knew his mind was so much better than his looks. Terry was shy, so it was hard for him to make friends. He knew if he were thinner, people would like him more. So

Terry decided to skip breakfast and dinner every day. Maybe if he lost weight, people would pay more attention to him instead of his SAT scores.

Kristy and Terry feel the way many teens feel. They think being thin will solve their problems. Once they're thin, Kristy and Terry are sure they will be accepted and make friends.

These two young people have a problem with low *self-esteem*. Self-esteem is how you feel about yourself. It is the feeling that you are likeable just the way you are. With high self-esteem you feel worthwhile, no matter what your size or shape.

There are certain times in life when self-esteem is more likely to be low. Adolescence (the teenage years) is one of those times. Adolescence is a time of many changes. It's common for teens to wonder if they are ready to grow up. It's normal to worry about how you look and what your peers (other teens) think of you.

It's also normal to feel bad about yourself every so often. Just remember that there are many things you can do to help yourself feel better. If you are overweight, that's nothing to be ashamed of. Weight problems are not easy to handle. You need to find someone who can help you plan the safest way to lose your unwanted pounds. Understanding more about your weight problem may also help you feel better about yourself. Reading this book is a great way to start.

What Is Fat?

Being fat means different things to different people. When someone says, "I'm fat," it could mean one of three things:

1. The person is *obese*.
   An obese person is very fat. He or she is more than 30 percent heavier than the ideal weight for his or her height. See the ideal weight chart on page 48.
2. The person is overweight.
   An overweight person is somewhat heavier than average.
3. The person "feels" fatter than he or she wants to be, even though his or her weight falls within the normal range.

"Fat" also has another meaning. It is one of the three major components of the food we eat. The other two are *carbohydrates* and *proteins*.

Fats come from milk products, meats, some fish, nuts, and vegetable oils. There is almost all fat in butter and margarine. Carbohydrates ("carbs") come from fruits, sugars, and foods made from flour (bread, pasta, crackers). Carbohydrates are the class of foods that supply energy to your body. Carbohydrates are also found in rice, corn, potatoes, and other vegetables. Protein is found in meat, fish, chicken, eggs, cheese, nuts, vegetables, and soybeans. Proteins are vital to the formation and activity of all living things.

We Need Body Fat

Fats are stored in cells called *adipocytes*. *Adipo-* means fat. *Cyte* means cell. Adipocytes cushion our organs and bones. They protect us from cold.

Fat cells also store *energy*. Energy is the ability of the body to do its work. Your body needs energy to grow. Energy makes your heart beat. It lets you blink your eyes and move your arms and legs.

You get energy from the foods you eat. *Calories* measure the amount of energy that each food produces when it is burned up by the body. If you eat more calories than you burn up, you gain weight. The excess weight is stored as fat.

Everyone is born with fat cells. Some people have too many. Extra cells develop during infancy and childhood. Some also develop during the teenage years. Once you stop growing, no new fat cells are added.

Unfortunately, once cells are added, they won't go away. But diet and exercise can help. It will not lower the total number of fat cells, but it can make each cell give up some of its fat and get smaller.

Why Am I Fat?

It's hard to tell at first why some people stay thin and others don't. Take, for example, Kim and Janey. They're both 15 and about 5'3" tall. They've got the same schedule of school classes and activities. They eat the same things at lunchtime. Yet Kim has a weight problem and Janey doesn't.

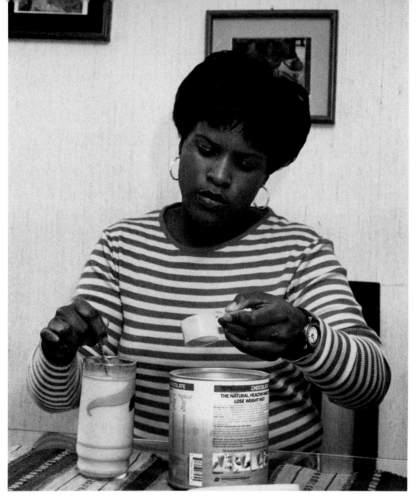

It is a good idea to check the nutritional value of any diet product.

It could be that Kim and Janey don't have the same *metabolism*. Metabolism is how your body operates and how much food it takes to give your body the energy it uses. Kim and Janey don't burn food at the same rate. Janey probably burns her food faster than Kim does.

It may be that Janey's body works differently than Kim's. Janey never sits still. She is always snapping her fingers and tapping her feet. Jane's extra body movements may use up more of her calories during the day.

Kim eats a sweet morning snack and nibbles on cookies before bedtime. Janey doesn't. These extra calories can add up to extra pounds.

Kim's mom is overweight. Her dad is stocky, with a large bone structure. Janey's parents are slim. Some researchers believe that the tendency to be fat can be passed on. They have found that a fat child usually has at least one fat parent. Some say that this shows that obesity is passed along in the genes. But other researchers disagree. They say that fat parents and children share the same poor eating habits. The overweight parent and child may also be somewhat inactive. Both eating and activity patterns will affect a family's weight.

Does your family eat small, lean meals and exercise regularly? Then you, like Janey, will probably not have a weight problem. If your family has not taught you good eating habits, you can learn them on your own.

What Is Right for Me?

You've probably seen charts giving the average height and weight for people of your age and sex. Remember that these figures are an average. Each person's "normal weight" or *set-point* differs. Your weight depends on your bone structure. It also depends on how much muscle development you have. You can actually be "overweight" on a chart without being fat. Take Les, for example. Les is a wrestler. He's developed lots of muscles. Muscle tissue is heavier than fat. If Les paid attention to the weight charts, he might think he's overweight. But he's not.

There are several ways doctors can measure body fat. A common, accurate method uses a special tool called a *skin-fold caliper.* The caliper gently squeezes and measures a fold of skin. Good places to measure are on the back and the upper arm. A thicker skin fold means more fat.

If you've been overweight since you were young, you probably carry around too many fat cells. Don't be discouraged. You can keep your weight down by keeping the level of fat in your cells low. But you can't keep your fat level low by *fad dieting.* Fad diets promote losing weight too quickly. You cannot stay on such a diet for a long time. As soon as you stop a fad diet, your "greedy" cells will grab onto all the extra calories your regular diet supplies. You'll gain back all the weight you lost—and fast!

The best way to keep your weight down is to learn how to make wise food choices. Learn how to cook low-fat meals. Learn how to enjoy healthy meals. Get in the habit of exercising. Then you will burn up calories *before* they are stored as fat.

If you've never had a weight problem, you may be worried about getting fat as you grow older. Now is the time to start good eating habits. These habits will become a way of life and will help you always to look and feel your best.

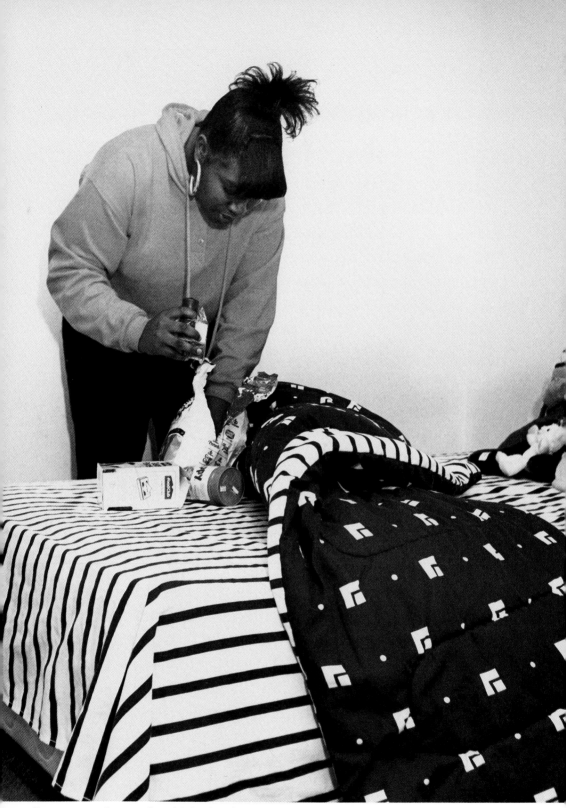

Some people need to hide food. Keeping a secret stash of food makes them feel secure.

Chapter 2

Causes of Overeating

Somehow in our society we've gotten the idea that people choose to be fat. We think that people are overweight because they lack willpower (self-control). We often think that if only they would make up their minds to eat less, they would be thin. Yet, many thin people will admit that they do not work to keep from gaining weight. Willpower alone does not determine how much people weigh.

Some people are able to avoid overeating. What if you're not one of these people? Does this mean you are weak or a failure? Certainly not! It may mean that you are overeating because you are unhappy. Or you may be a *compulsive eater*. This is a person who cannot resist eating. Feelings deep inside force compulsive eaters to overeat. The problem is that compulsive eaters don't always eat because they are hungry.

Sometimes people overeat just to have some-thing to do with their hands. Snacking is common while watching television or a movie. Some other reasons why people eat more than they should are:

- to reward themselves
- to please others
- to avoid waste, especially at restaurants
- to be a good guest.

What You Learned as a Child

For most people, eating is also a social function. Little babies first experience loving human contact through eating. They are cuddled and comforted when they eat. Many children never lose this feel-ing that food is soothing, even after they have grown up. Mealtimes can be a time for family sharing. Parties and holiday celebrations are often arranged around food. It's easy to overeat when so many of your favorite foods have been prepared. Relatives may expect you to sample all of their special dishes. Family members may feel loved when you eat the food they prepare.

For some children, eating may be a way to deal with their problems. Have you ever "pigged out" because you felt sad, depressed, lonely, nervous, or angry? Usually, eating can make you feel better for a time. Unfortunately, it doesn't help you to under-stand what caused the negative feelings. In fact, overeating may actually cause another problem: guilt.

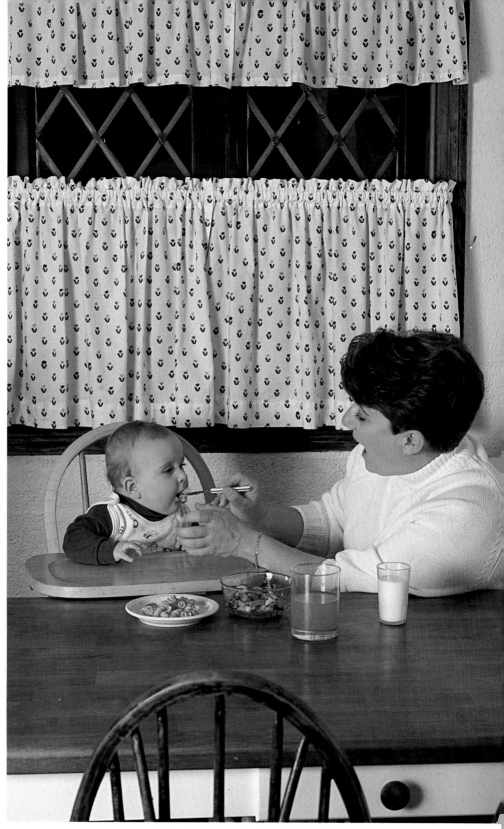

Attitudes about food and eating are formed at an early age.

Clarice often felt guilty about overeating. She knew she was the biggest girl in her class. Whenever she looked in the mirror, all she could see were fat hips, feet that were too wide, and arms that were plump. Whenever she had a bad day, she ate more. The more she ate, the fatter Clarice felt.

How can Clarice continue to overeat when it makes her feel so fat and unattractive? Clarice is caught in a *cycle* of overeating. Even though she is unhappy with the way she looks, she uses food to make herself feel better. Her overeating then makes her feel guilty. Clarice, like most teens, is critical of herself. You may have had similar feelings. You may find it hard to focus on your good points. You may only see what you don't like.

Are You Too Hard on Yourself?

Have you stopped to think where your critical thoughts come from? Perhaps your parents are overworked and busy. They don't pay much attention to you. You may be feeling unloved. You may think that you have done something to upset them. You may think you can change this unhappy situation by "being better." To you, "being better" may mean being thinner and more attractive.

Perhaps you have relatives or friends who are very critical. Maybe you've grown up with the feeling that you're not as great as you "should be." Or perhaps you have set standards for yourself that are too tough. Maybe you compare yourself to the wrong people. You put yourself down for not being as popular or attractive as they are.

This kind of judging and comparing goes on all the time. No one person can truly judge another. Who's to say what's really "attractive" or "the best"? It's hard to fight off critical feelings if you don't feel good about your body. Your *body image* is how satisfied you are with your size and shape. It is changeable. When you're feeling "up," your body image is great. When you're feeling "down," your body image will most likely be low.

You probably have in your mind a picture of the perfect body. You know just how you would look if you could make yourself over. These ideas come mainly from three places:

- your peers
- your parents
- the media (television, newspapers, magazines, and movies).

Each group has their own opinions about how you should look. Usually the message is that being thin is fashionable and healthy.

What Society Has to Say

"Thin" hasn't always been "in." Look at a painting by the Flemish artist Rubens, or the Italian master Titian. Most of the people shown in their art are plump. The women are full-figured. In

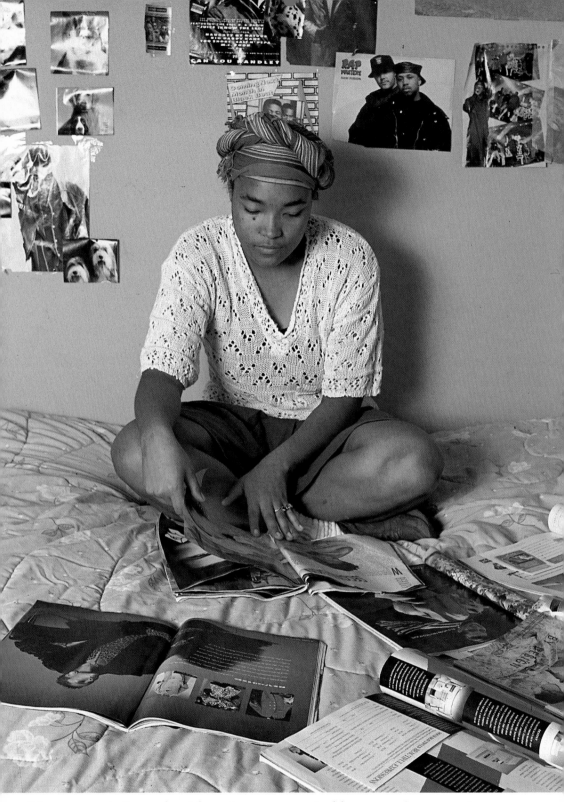

Many expectations about beauty are promoted by magazines, movies, and television.

American society around the 1900s, plump women were also thought to be more attractive than skinny ones.

Even now, in some cultures, fat is respected. In Japan, sumo wrestlers are highly honored. They are huge men with large waists. They must continually overeat to maintain their size. In many poorer countries today, people want to be fat. This is a sign that they are wealthy. They are proud to be able to afford as much food as they want.

Today in America, however, fat is considered ugly. Overeating is considered unwise, unhealthy, and sometimes unforgivable.

If you are overweight, or think you are, this can put a lot of pressure on you. The more ads you see, the more stress you may feel. You may think that you've got to eat the right foods and drink the right drinks. You may think that more people will love you if you could only be thin. If you believe that being thin will make you happy and improve your self-esteem, you're likely to try just about any new fad diet that comes along. It is true that losing weight and getting into shape can often make you feel better about yourself. But you should be aware of who is causing you to become thinner. Is it truly your own desire, or are you doing it because you feel pressure from others?

Remember, there are healthy and unhealthy ways to lose weight. In the following chapter you will learn how to make good choices for yourself.

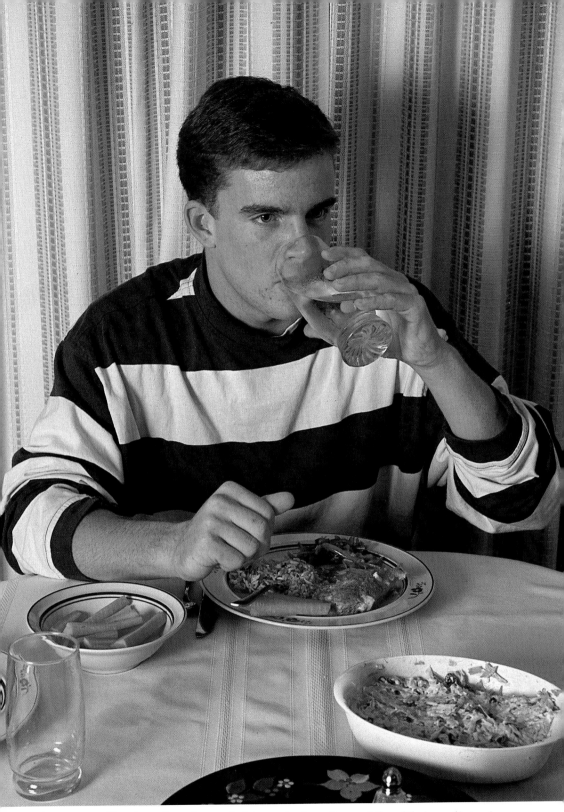

The most effective plan for weight control and good health is a diet of low-fat foods and reasonable portions.

Chapter 3

The Dangers of Diet Fads

"Lose twenty pounds in two weeks!"

"How to look your best in ten easy steps!"

"Get thin without ever feeling hungry!"

These are the kinds of ads you read in today's fashion magazines and hear on television. Americans spend millions each year searching for the "perfect diet." But many people are wasting their money. There is no magic plan that will make fat disappear quickly and permanently.

Some diet plans have been successful. Others have not. Some have proved to be dangerous.

If fad diets can be so harmful, why do people spend money on them? Many people feel hopeless about their weight and appearance. They're willing to do almost anything to get help. A fad diet looks like a quick solution to their problems.

With any weight reduction program it's hard to *keep* the weight off. More than 85 percent of all dieters regain their lost weight in two years. The body is used to processing food for a fatter person. Dieters often find themselves slipping back to their old eating habits. The result is a "yo-yo" effect. A lot of weight is lost fast. But a lot of weight is gained back quickly. The person feels guilty and starts a new diet. The yo-yo cycle continues.

Such a cycle of gaining and losing weight is dangerous. It's more of a strain on the body than staying at one level, even an overweight level. Yo-yo dieting tends to raise the fat and cholesterol levels in the blood. This increases the risk of heart disease.

Have you thought about trying one of these so-called "miracle diets"? Before you do, consider the harm they might cause your body.

Fasting

Fasting is a time when a person does not eat, or eats very little. Sometimes people fast for religious purposes. But this is usually for a short time, a few hours or a single day. Fasting for longer periods of time is not a healthy way to lose weight. It deprives your body of important minerals known as *electrolytes*. Electrolytes send an electrical message that causes the heart to beat correctly. By fasting, you may develop dangerous heart problems even if you do not have a history of heart trouble.

Low-Carbohydrate Diets

These diets are based on eating few carbohydrates (breads, starches, pasta). Instead of the high-energy foods, the dieter eats lots of eggs, meat, chicken, fish, cheese, and other high-protein foods. These foods are also high in fats and cholesterol that can lead to heart problems in some people. Other side effects of a low-carbohydrate diet may be:

- bad breath
- headaches
- fainting
- dehydration (losing too much water)
- cravings for carbohydrates, especially candy.

If a dieter gives in to the craving for candy, the extra calories will not help to lose weight!

Liquid Diets

Most liquid diets suggest a diet drink for two meals. Only one meal allows solid food. Special foods may be part of the diet plan, too.

Many people have success with liquid diets—at first. But it's hard to live on diet drinks for long periods of time. Once off the liquid diet, the dieter doesn't know how to make sensible meal choices. It is easy to go back to the old eating habits and regain the lost weight.

Liquid diet programs can be expensive. Most of these programs are supposed to be done with the help of a doctor or other health professional. Unfortunately, teens on liquid diets tend to buy the products at drug stores. They don't work with a doctor or nutritionist. Many teens use the products incorrectly and suffer side effects such as:

- nausea
- dizziness
- extreme fatigue
- hair loss
- irritability
- irregular menstruation (periods).

Diet Pills

The most powerful diet pills available contain *amphetamines.* Amphetamines must be prescribed by a doctor. These drugs "pep up" the body and decrease appetite. They only work for a short time and are very dangerous if used incorrectly. Large amounts of amphetamines over time may cause permanent brain damage, extreme fatigue, and even death. Amphetamines are powerful drugs.

Other diet pills are sold without a doctor's prescription. They are well advertised on television and at drug stores. Many of these pills use sugar to control appetite. Unfortunately, the sugar adds extra calories.

Some diet pills are *diuretics* (drugs that make the body lose water). Diuretics don't make you lose fat. They can be dangerous if misused. The body needs water to remain healthy.

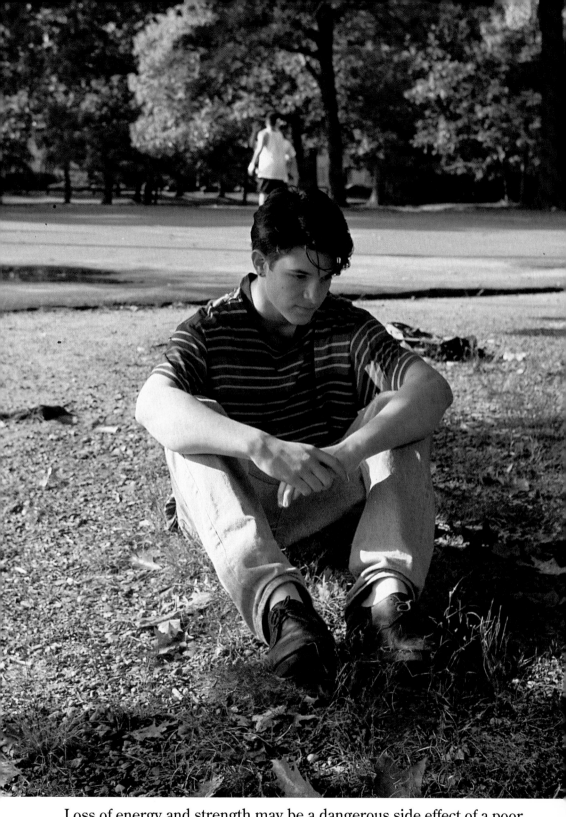

Loss of energy and strength may be a dangerous side effect of a poor diet plan.

Laxatives

Drugs that cause bowel movements are known as laxatives. Sometimes dieters use them to rid, or *purge*, the body of unwanted food. Unfortunately, many important vitamins and minerals may also be lost this way.

Overuse of laxatives can cause abdominal (stomach) pain, cramps, and diarrhea. Overuse of laxatives may also cause extreme fatigue. The body has no energy to function.

Laxatives should only be used for occasional irregularity. If you use laxatives to diet, your body will begin to depend on them. Once you stop using them, it may be difficult to have a bowel movement normally.

Anorexia Nervosa

Anorexia nervosa is an eating disorder that causes extreme thinness due to self-starvation. Healthy teens need anywhere from 1,200 to 3,000 calories a day. *Anorectics* (persons with anorexia) may eat as little as 300 to 600 calories a day.

Most anorectics are young women ages 13 to 19. They seem to have some things in common. Many come from fairly well-to-do families. Anorectics try to please everyone. They never feel quite good enough or thin enough. Anorectics try to solve their problems by starving themselves. In this way, they control at least one part of their lives—their diet. Their minds are taken over by thoughts of

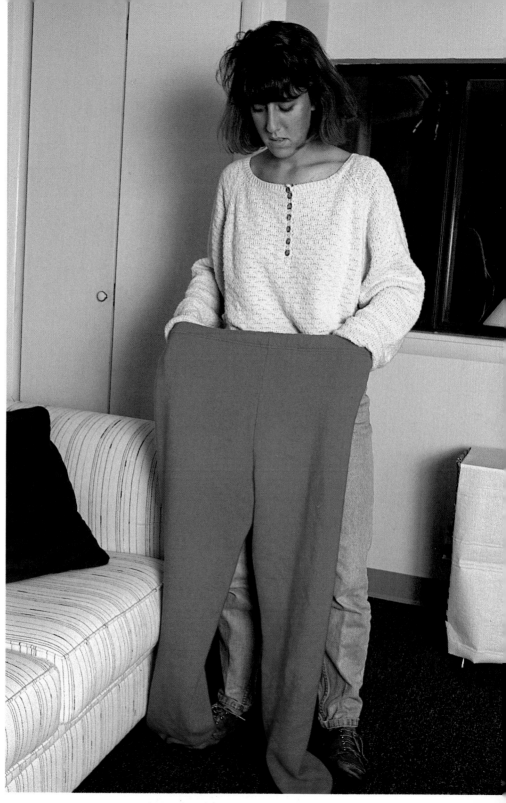

It is not healthy for the body to go through drastic cycles of weight loss and weight gain.

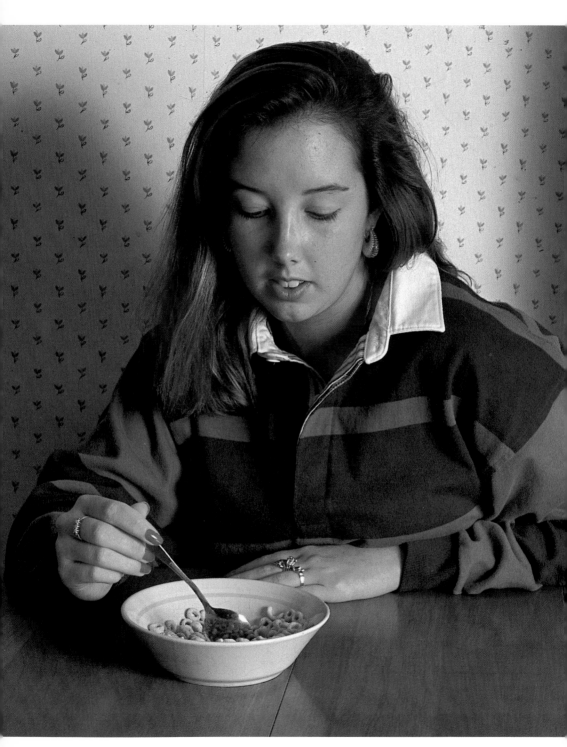

Anorectics may just pick at food or refuse to eat anything.

food. Anorectics see themselves as fat, even though they are extremely thin.

Anorectics develop strange eating habits. For example, each piece of food might be cut in a set number of pieces or chewed an exact number of times. Meals can become tense and uncomfortable for everyone when an anorectic is at the table.

Some side effects of anorexia are:
- dry skin
- dull, brittle hair that falls out
- constipation
- mental confusion
- disturbed sleep
- icy hands and feet
- downy fuzz on face, body, and limbs
- loss of muscle and fat
- loss of menstrual periods in females.

Anorectics may starve themselves until they weigh as little as 60 or 70 pounds. They look like skeletons covered with skin. Many times hospitalization is necessary. Even with treatment, as many as 20 percent starve themselves to death.

Bulimia

Bulimia means "abnormal hunger." It is an eating disorder known as the "binge-purge syndrome." A *bulimic* (someone with bulimia) gorges, or binges, on huge amounts of food. He or she then gets rid of the food by vomiting or using laxatives. Diuretics and diet pills may also be used.

Bulimics crave food, especially high-fat, high-sugar foods. The cravings, however, do not come from hunger. They are caused by emotional problems. Like anorectics, bulimics don't feel good about themselves. Some get started bingeing and purging because their friends do it to lose weight. Bulimia is harder to diagnose than anorexia, because bulimics often look normal. Binge-purge cycles have many unhealthy side effects:

- loss of tooth enamel from repeated vomiting
- sores and scar tissue on the esophagus (food tube)
- swollen glands in the neck under the jaw
- loss of important vitamins and minerals
- indigestion, cramps, and constipation
- possible kidney damage or heart problems.

Bulimics usually feel ashamed about their vomiting. They are afraid of being discovered. They often withdraw from family and friends.

Health Foods

All foods promoted as "health" or "natural" foods may not be wise diet choices. Oatmeal muffins contain oat bran, a good source of fiber. But many muffins have more calories and fat than cream-filled doughnuts. Some fruit-filled yogurts can be high in sugar. Check the labels of the foods you buy. It is important to know what you are eating even if you are not on a diet.

Vegetarian Diets

A diet without meat can be healthful if practiced with good sense. A balance of important vitamins and minerals is necessary. Such a balance can only be obtained by careful meal planning.

Even vegetarian diets have fad versions. Some diet plans eliminate all fish, poultry, and dairy products as well as meat. This is often not a wise diet for teens. By avoiding so many important food groups, it's hard to take in enough protein and calcium for normal growth. This type of diet also tends to be low in vitamin B_{12}, which may cause skin problems, diarrhea, and mental confusion.

Choosing a Safe Diet

Check with your doctor and your parents before starting any diet. Nutritionists recommend losing no more than one pound a week. A sensible diet should include:

- a variety of nutritious foods
- few high-calorie items (candy and desserts)
- sufficient protein
- enough carbohydrates (breads and pasta)
- lots of vegetables and fruits
- small amounts of fat (butter, oils, fatty meats).

You don't need to take on too rigid a diet. If it's too tough, you probably won't follow it for long. It is best to have a long-term plan for weight loss that you can live with.

DAILY FOOD GUIDE

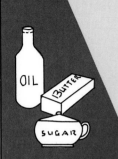

Fats, Oils, and Sweets

USE SPARINGLY

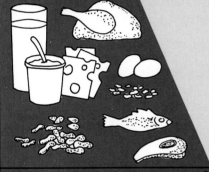

Milk, Yogurt, Eggs, Cheeses,
Meat, Fish, Dry Beans,
and Nuts

2–3 SERVINGS

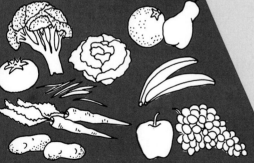

Vegetables and Fruits

3–5 SERVINGS

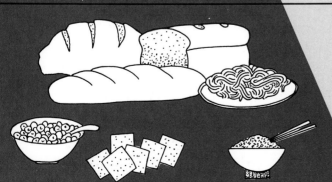

Bread, Rice,
Cereal, and
Pasta

**6–11
SERVINGS**

Sources: U.S. Department of Agriculture. U.S. Department of Health and Human Services.

You can avoid diets that require you to buy many special products. Pre-packaged diet foods are expensive. It is possible to lose weight and stay healthy by eating regular foods. You need to do some meal planning before you shop. And you should try to buy only what you need for your plan at the supermarket. Then you won't be tempted to grab the wrong foods at home when you are hungry.

Many people shed weight quickly in the first week or two. Then their weight loss levels off. Much of the first weight lost is water. Some people try to increase their weight loss by taking diuretics. This is not wise. Remember, diuretics do nothing to reduce fat. They cause the body to lose important vitamins and minerals.

A Diet Summary

As you have learned, *a good diet is based on healthy eating habits.* Once you've lost your desired amount of weight, you should continue with the same healthy eating habits. Then the weight lost will most likely stay off.

Fad diets over a period of time are clearly dangerous. They harm both the body and the mind. They can lead to life-threatening eating disorders such as anorexia nervosa and bulimia. Avoid *any* diet that promises a large weight loss in a short time. Use the suggestions in this book to break the cycle of overeating and develop your own plan for healthy eating.

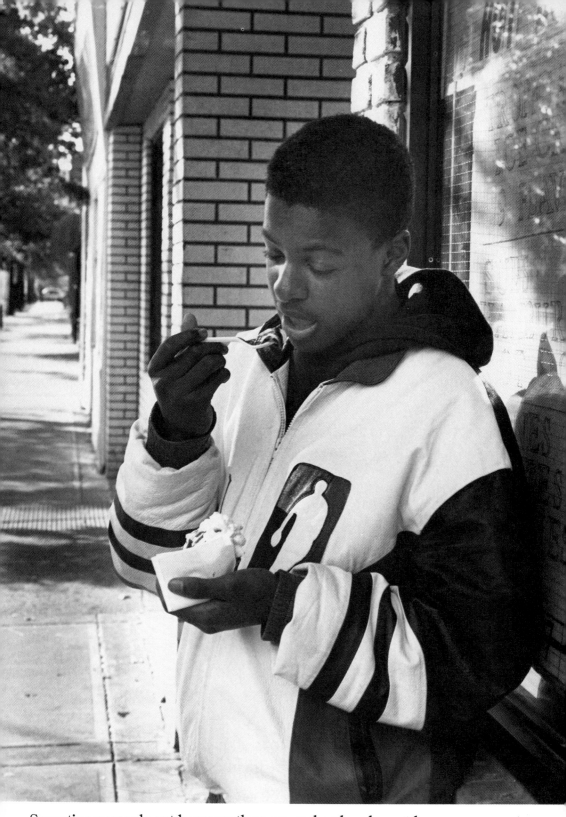

Sometimes people eat because they are sad or lonely, not because they are really hungry.

Chapter 4

Understanding Hunger

Fourteen-year-old Chelsea tells this story:

"My twin brothers were always getting into trouble. I hated to listen to my parents yelling at them. So I tried to be 'the good girl.' I always did just what I was told. I pretended that everything about my life was just great. But deep inside I knew I had problems. I found that I always felt better after eating. So I began to eat more and more. It didn't matter what I ate; it was a way to shut out my bad feelings."

Chelsea lost her ability to make sensible choices about eating. She didn't eat when she was hungry. She ate to feel better. Chelsea's eating habits are poor, but not uncommon. Eating for her is more than a way to satisfy nutritional needs. Food fills an *emotional* need. It comforts her.

A Creature of Habit

Certain activities and feelings lead to food choices that are based on habit, not hunger. For some, coming home from school means eating a sweet snack. For others, going to a friend's house means it's time for munchies. Watching television can be a signal to bring out the ice cream. People with weight problems often make these kinds of choices—almost without thinking.

Television ads may foster bad eating habits. Food is shown and talked about so much that it can make you feel everyone else is eating and having fun. You join in, many times, even though you aren't hungry.

It's OK to have snacks on occasion. And it's great to enjoy good food in the company of friends. The problem is that too often we eat without thinking. We need to be aware of *why* we are eating.

If you're overweight, think of how you are feeling when you have the desire to eat. If you cannot control your food intake, you may need help for some emotional problem. In time it may feel more natural to choose non-eating activities when you are upset. You'll be on your way to developing new, healthier habits.

Why Do You Eat?

Do you eat when you are afraid or lonely? Do you eat when you are frustrated? Do you tell yourself, "I'm so fat. I might as well go ahead and eat.

What difference does it make?" Once you understand your reasons for eating, you'll be better able to control your eating. Here's a plan to help you get started:

1. Write down your reasons for overeating. Be honest with yourself. Do this in a quiet place. What you write is private.
2. Write down your reasons for wanting to lose weight. Look closely at what you've written. Are these *your* reasons? Or have you written down what you think others expect of you?
3. Write down what makes you feel good about yourself. There is something about you that makes you special. These thoughts will help you feel "up" when you're tempted to overeat.
4. Make an eating chart. Write down everything you eat for each meal and snack. Also include:

   - when you eat
   - where you eat
   - whom you eat with
   - how you feel at the time.

Keep this chart for two weeks. With it, you can learn many things about yourself. It will show you when you make eating choices based on feelings, instead of true hunger.

Learn to Recognize Hunger

Your stomach and brain give you signals about when and how much to eat. The signals are related

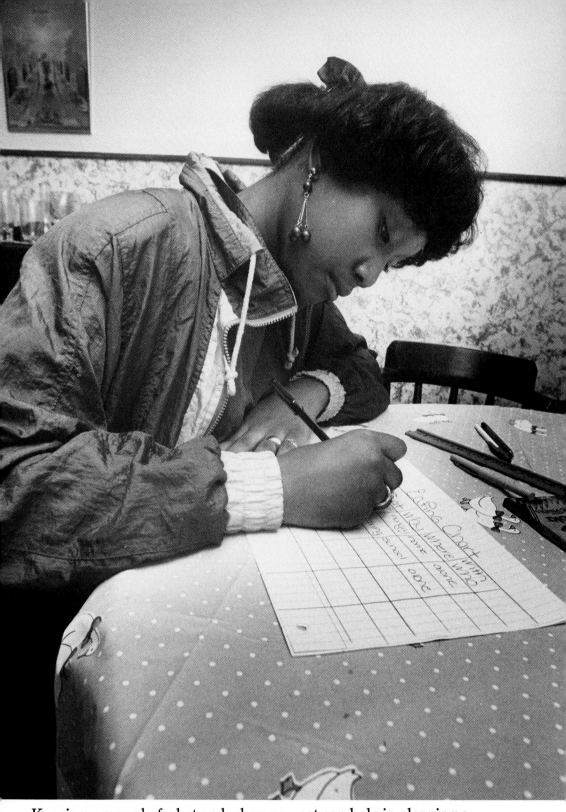

Keeping a record of what and when you eat can help in planning a sensible weight-loss program.

to your blood sugar levels. Blood sugar carries fuel to the cells. It stays at a certain level a few hours after a meal. When you eat something sweet, your blood sugar level rises. It also rises after a large meal. It drops during exercise and activity. As it drops, your stomach may "growl." This is a sign of hunger.

For each person, blood sugar enters the muscles at a different rate. The rate depends on how active you are and how much body fat you have. You probably know thin people who always seem to be snacking. Yet they never gain weight. They eat just enough food to satisfy their hunger. Their blood sugar stays at about the same level all the time.

Let's look at what can happen to blood sugar levels during a typical day. This will help you understand how to recognize true hunger pangs.

When you get up in the morning, your blood sugar level depends on what you ate the night before. If you ate half a pizza at midnight, you may not feel hungry right away. As you rush about getting ready for the day, you use up a lot of blood sugar. You'll start to feel hungry. If you don't eat, you may get a headache. You may even feel faint, dizzy, or sick to your stomach.

If you ignore these hunger signals, your blood sugar will remain low. Your body will slow down to save energy. You may begin to feel sleepy and find it hard to concentrate.

Your liver will then send signals to increase your blood sugar level. Suddenly, you'll pep up. Lots of people think this means they don't need to eat during the day. Some people trick their bodies into getting this full feeling. This is done by drinking caffeine drinks such as coffee, tea, or soda.

Going without food or living on caffeine is a strain on your system. When you finally eat, your body holds on to more of the calories. It won't use up any of your stored fat.

There is another problem with trying to go without food. By the end of the day, you're starving. Studies have shown that people who wait all day to eat actually eat *more* in 24 hours because their hunger is so huge. In fact, some people who skip a meal end up eating twice as much at the next meal.

If you want to lose weight, listen to your body. Pay attention to your blood sugar signals. If your stomach is growling, eat something healthy. You may not need much. Try some fruit and cheese. Avoid sugary foods with "empty calories" that will send your blood sugar level up fast and high, but not for long. When it drops back down again, you may feel even more hungry than before. It is always better to choose healthy foods that will satisfy your hunger longer. This way you will probably end up eating less in the long run.

Chapter 5

Positive Planning

You probably have a mental picture of yourself. It is made up of the thoughts you tell yourself over and over. Often these thoughts are negative. For example, you may tell yourself:

"I'm fat and unattractive."

"I can't change."

"I've got no willpower."

"I'll never be thin, I've got big bones."

If you think negative thoughts long enough, you can be trapped into believing them. But you can break out of this trap. Think ahead to what you *want* to be. Form a new picture of yourself in your mind. A positive self-image may help you to reach your goals for self-improvement.

Be realistic. You won't be able to make all the changes at once.

Write down your own goals on a "New Me" form. Complete the following statements:

My ideal weight is _____.

To reach my ideal weight I will change my eating habits by not _____.

At my new weight, I will try to do these things differently: _____.

If I stray from my diet plan sometimes, I will

_____.

Often, our most negative thoughts are about dieting itself. Think about the advertising you may have heard for diet plans. Maybe they promise things like:

- Lose 50 pounds fast!
- The more weight you lose, the better you'll feel!
- Don't eat all weekend and feel great!
- You only need one meal a day!

These diet statements are unhealthy and dangerous. They are also hard to achieve. Plan a healthy diet that is manageable. Remember that no one is perfect . On some meals, you will "cheat" a little. That's normal. Think about what you've done right with your diet, not what you couldn't resist. At bedtime each day, remind yourself that you did your best, and tomorrow you can do even better.

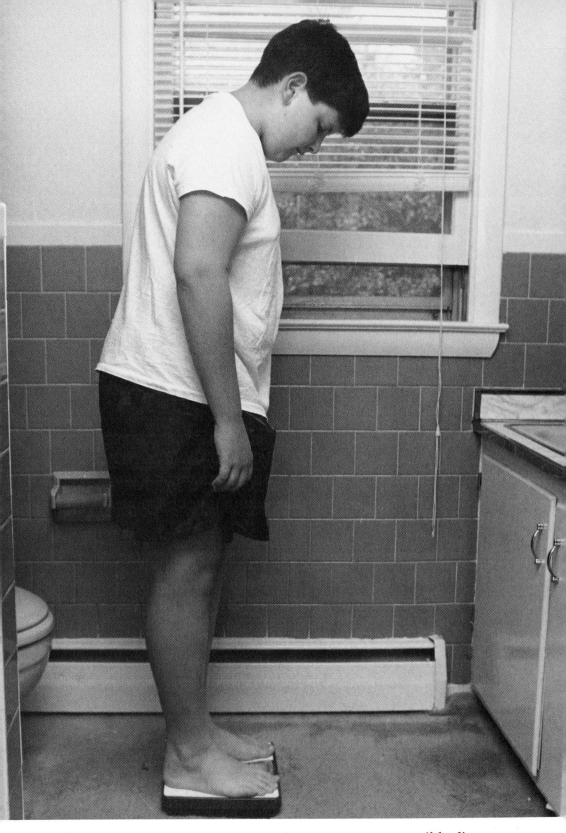

Regular weighing can track steady progress on a sensible diet.

Calorie Count

Think positively about what you *can* eat instead of what you *can't*. Calories are only a problem if you take in more than you burn up. Look at the chart below. It shows the recommended amount of calories teens need to maintain their ideal weight.

TOTAL CALORIES NEEDED TO MAINTAIN IDEAL WEIGHT				
		Male		
HEIGHT	IDEAL WEIGHT	INACTIVE	ACTIVE	VERY ACTIVE
5'6"	142	1,562	2,130	2,556
5'7"	148	1,628	2,220	2,664
5'8"	154	1,694	2,310	2,772
5'9"	160	1,760	2,400	2,880
5'10"	166	1,826	2,490	2,988
5'11"	172	1,892	2,580	3,096
6'0"	178	1,958	2,670	3,204
6'1"	184	2,024	2,760	3,312
6'2"	190	2,090	2,850	3,420
6'3"	196	2,156	2,940	3,528
6'4"	202	2,222	3,030	3,636
		Female		
HEIGHT	IDEAL WEIGHT	INACTIVE	ACTIVE	VERY ACTIVE
5'0"	100	1,100	1,500	1,800
5'1"	105	1,155	1,575	1,890
5'2"	110	1,210	1,650	1,980
5'3"	115	1,265	1,725	2,070
5'4"	120	1,320	1,800	2,160
5'5"	125	1,375	1,875	2,250
5'6"	130	1,430	1,950	2,340
5'7"	135	1,485	2,025	2,430
5'8"	140	1,540	2,100	2,520
5'9"	145	1,595	2,175	2,610
5'10"	150	1,650	2,250	2,700

Fat Count

Reducing fat in your diet is one of the best ways to improve your health and to lose weight. There are different kinds of fats in different kinds of foods. Meats and cheeses, for example, contain animal fats. Olive oil and peanut butter contain vegetable fats. In general, animal fats are not as desirable as vegetable fats. Animal fats are often high in cholesterol. Vegetable fats are not. For almost any food product you buy, information about fat, calories, and cholesterol is listed on the packaging along with ingredients and other nutritional data. You don't have to avoid *all* fat entirely to diet successfully. Experts suggest, as a general rule, that a healthy diet consists of foods that get no more than 30 percent of their calories from fat. That means less than one-third of all the calories you consume should be from fat.

Lifelong Diet Planning

The chart on page 36 is a summary of basic food groups and suggested number of servings. If you are very active or still growing, you'll need to allow for more calories. Ask your doctor or nutritionist for more information on food groups and calorie counts for specific foods in each category. Then you can keep track of your daily calories, and adjust your number of servings.

To help you keep track of your allowed foods, draw a daily chart. After each meal, check off what you have eaten. Another way is to cut strips of paper. Write each allowed food on a strip. Store the strips on one side of a notebook. As you eat the food, move the strip for that food to the other side of the notebook. By the end of the day, you should have moved all your strips to the other side.

Watch Out for Hidden Calories

Most people think of a salad as a low-calorie meal. Salads can be a healthy diet choice with some exceptions. Watch out for the high-fat, high-calorie extras. Avoid too much cheese, avocado, bacon bits, garbanzo beans, and fatty dressings. You can eat as much lettuce, cucumber, celery, onions, mushrooms, and alfalfa sprouts as you want. These veggies have virtually no calories.

How much soda do you drink daily? Soda contains no vitamins or minerals necessary for good health. But a 12-ounce can of regular soda has 9 teaspoons of sugar. Sometimes so-called sugar-free soda contains corn syrup or other sweeteners. Read the labels to make sure you're getting a true low-calorie product. It is important to drink a lot of fluids each day. But an even better drink than soda is vegetable juice or low-fat or non-fat (skim) milk. It is also a good idea to drink at least eight glasses of water a day.

Chapter 6

Diet Tips for Good Eating Habits

Deciding to make healthy food choices is easier said than done, but it's worth it. As you learn new eating habits and lose weight, your self-image will change. You'll feel better about yourself. Here are some practical hints for success:

When you're tempted to snack, *do* something.

Get up and go for a walk. (Do not walk to the refrigerator!) Call a friend. Do a load of laundry. Write a letter. Do some yard work. Research has shown that the urge to eat usually dies down after 20 minutes. Try to keep busy for at least 20 minutes. A drink of water may be enough to satisfy you after that.

51

Make an emergency box to keep in the refrigerator.

Fill it with carrots, celery, broccoli, green peppers, and tomatoes. When you get the irresistible urge to snack, head for your emergency box instead of a candy box!

Change your eating style.

Chew more slowly. Be sure to swallow between each bite. These suggestions sound obvious. But think about them during your next meal. Check to see if you're gulping down your food. If you are, slow down and taste your food. Eating with others can also help. If you stop to talk or listen during meals, you will naturally eat more slowly.

Pause in the middle of a meal. Make a point of carrying on a conversation. (It's tough to talk with your mouth full!)

When you're eating, just eat. Don't read. Don't talk on the phone. Don't watch TV. Concentrate on the textures and smells of what you're eating. Take the time to enjoy each meal and snack.

Quit the "clean plate" club.

Leave a little bit on your plate at the end of each meal. You may have to persuade your family to allow this. Explain that you're trying to break yourself of the habit of overeating.

Get rid of temptation.

Have you got cookies stashed in your desk drawer? Does your family have a candy dish in

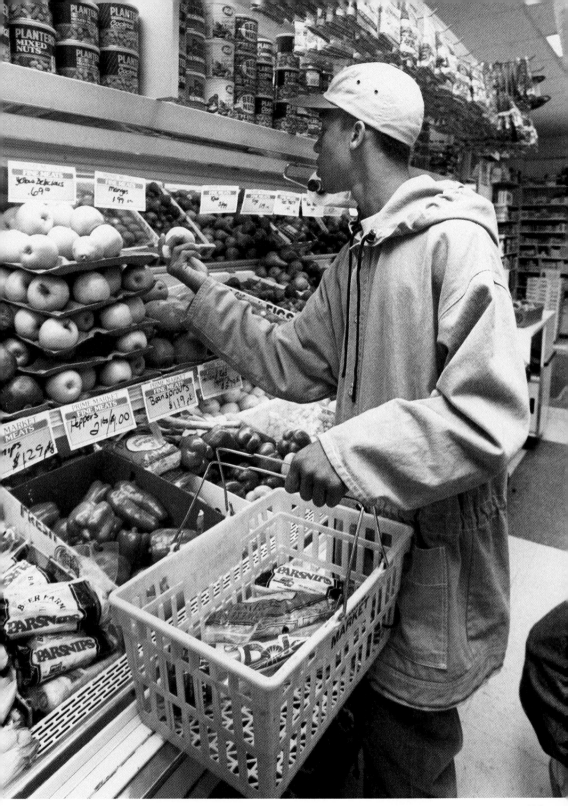

Fresh fruits and vegetables are good snacks and add
important nutritional value to a diet.

almost every room? What goodies are in the
backseat of the car? Ask your family's help in keeping all food in the kitchen only.

Plan your snacks and meals.

Begin with one meal at a time. For example, set
limits before going to a restaurant. Tell yourself:

"I can drink water instead of a soft drink."

"I will avoid high-fat foods.

"I'll have fruit at home for my dessert."

Thinking through choices ahead of time will
help you avoid the temptation to overeat. This is
especially important when you're going out with
friends.

Look for low-fat foods.

The American diet tends to be full of high-fat,
high-calorie foods. Examples are red meats, chips
and dips, gravies, cream sauces, cheeses, and desserts. The average fast-food meal gets about 50
percent of its calories from fat. (The Japanese diet
is only 15 percent fat.) Eating lots of high-fat food
may lead to heart disease.

Some suggestions for how to limit your fat
intake are to:

- eat more fish and skinless chicken or turkey
- choose pizza with whole grain crust and
  vegetable toppings
- try baking or broiling foods instead of frying
- try stir-frying, which requires only a little oil
  to cook.

Use your scale wisely.

Don't weigh yourself every day. It's too soon to see any changes. Instead, weigh yourself once a week at the same time of the day.

Reward yourself!

If you've reached your goal for the week, treat yourself to something special. Go to a movie. Buy a new book. Praise yourself for doing well.

One of the best rewards for people watching their weight is food. Pick a favorite food. Allow yourself a reasonable amount of it. You'll have this reward to look forward to for each week of dieting. For example, a scoop of your favorite ice cream makes a great reward. But make it a single scoop!

Add exercise.

Your natural weight is a kind of balance between the daily calories taken in and the calories used up. In order to reduce weight, a body needs to burn up more calories than it takes in.

Researchers have found that total weight loss is greater and healthier when dieters exercise. The more you move, the more calories you burn. Therefore, the more you exercise, the more you can eat. Think of the variety of foods you can enjoy—maybe even dessert once in a while.

With regular exercise, your appetite will decrease. Exercise also helps your body use food more efficiently. This means your body will need less food each day.

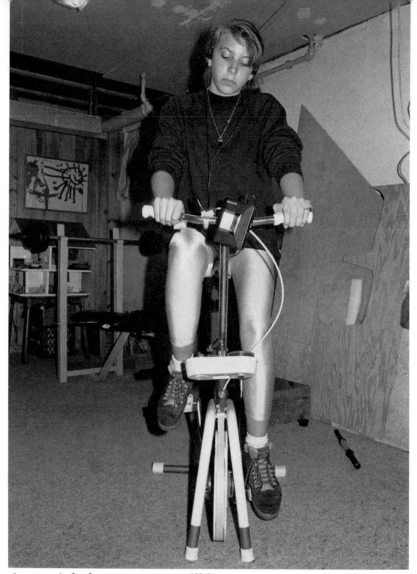
Any weight-loss program will be improved by regular exercise.

Exercise also helps us deal with *stress.* Stress is the body's way of showing that a change has taken place. Not all stress is bad. Getting a special award causes a good kind of stress. Failing a test is not so good. When your body is fit, it handles stress better. If you feel less stressed, it is also true that you might not need to make those extra trips to the refrigerator.

Another good thing about exercise is that it increases energy levels. Right after exercising, you may feel a bit tired. But with regular exercise, you will have more energy throughout the day.

Exercise will also build up and define your muscles. Muscle tissue weighs more than fat. But don't be discouraged. Fortunately, toned muscles look a whole lot better than fat!

No Excuses

Many overweight people are sensitive about their looks. This sensitivity makes it hard for them to try public activities such as swimming, team sports, or dancing. If you've been overweight all your life, you may never have been active. But even if you haven't learned these skills, you can develop a successful exercise program at home.

Remember that the exercise is for *you*, not someone else. You can start by working out in private just a few minutes a day. Try stretching exercises. They're not strenuous. Stretching will help you use up calories. It can also firm up your muscles. Try running in place or riding a stationary bike. Doing these activities while watching television may help make time pass faster. Begin slowly. You may need help to design a program that is right for you. Ask your gym teacher how to get started.

Perhaps you've avoided exercise because you're not competitive. Were you always the last one to be picked for team sports at school? Do you find that you don't really care whether you come in first or last? You don't need to be competitive to exercise. All you need is the desire to "work" your body. Try walking. Join a beginning dance or exercise class. If you're with others who are also learning new skills, you'll feel more comfortable.

Perhaps you're thinking, "I don't have time to exercise." Many people feel that way. But there are hidden opportunities for exercise during daily activities. Stretch while talking on the phone. Tighten muscles in your buttocks while you sit in class or ride in a car. Whatever you're doing, ask yourself, "Is this the most energetic way I can do this?" For example, whenever you can:

- take the stairs instead of the elevator
- stand instead of sit
- walk instead of ride
- run instead of walk.

How much time should you exercise daily? Set a realistic goal, especially if you haven't been exercising regularly. Doctors suggest that you build up to at least 15-20 minutes of vigorous exercise daily. Or that you do 30 minutes of vigorous exercise every other day.

Pick something you *like* to do. That way, you will have a better chance of staying with your program. Make exercise something you look forward to doing each day.

A Lifetime of Healthy Eating

Changing any habit is hard work. It is especially hard if you try to make lots of changes at once. This is certainly true for developing new healthy eating habits. These are some of the strongest habits in your daily life.

Be patient with yourself. You'll still make some poor food choices. You'll overeat on occasion. You're human. Forgive yourself and get back to your diet plan.

Unfortunately, no one has found an easy way to lose weight and keep it off. Weight loss is not a simple matter. You are not alone, however. There are many people willing to help you. Look on page 61 for some organizations that can help.

Some days you'll feel that you can tackle your weight problem easily. Other days you may feel discouraged and angry. These feelings are normal. But you *can* learn to deal with a weight problem. When you can make sensible and healthy eating choices, you will like the results. Give yourself time. There are no quick solutions, no "magic" diets. There are only hard work and determination. Ask the people you know who have reached their diet goals. They will be happy to tell you what worked for them. Give it a try—what have you got to lose but some weight?

Glossary—*Explaining New Words*

adolescence The years that begin at puberty (about age 10-12) and end when the body stops growing (about age 18-20).

amphetamines Drugs that speed up the functions of the brain and body.

anorexia nervosa An eating disorder that results in severe weight loss; self-starvation.

bingeing Eating an unusually large amount of food in a short time.

bulimia An eating disorder that establishes a cycle of bingeing and purging.

calorie A unit of measure for the amount of energy our bodies get from food.

compulsive eater One who cannot resist eating.

diuretics Drugs that cause the body to eliminate water by increasing the flow of urine.

energy Body's ability to do work.

fad or **crash diet** A diet that promises quick weight loss by limiting the number of foods or food groups.

fasting Period of time during which someone chooses not to eat.

laxatives Drugs that cause bowel movements.

purging Getting rid of unwanted food by dangerous methods such as intentional vomiting.

self-image How we feel about ourselves.

set-point The body's "natural" weight.

stress The body's way of showing a change has taken place.

Where to Get Help

You may want to talk with someone you know and trust about good eating habits and healthy ways to lose weight. He or she may support you while you are following your new diet program. You may also want to call or write:

**President's Council on Physical Fitness
   and Sports**
Department of Health and Human Services
450 5th Street, Suite 7103
Washington, D.C. 20001
202-272-3430
Free publications are available on many aspects of physical fitness.

Consumer Information Center
P.O. Box 100
Pueblo, CO 81002
This agency can provide free publications on exercise, weight control, and good nutrition.

**National Association of Anorexia Nervosa
   and Associate Disorders (ANAD)**
Box 7
Highland Park, IL 60035
708-831-3438
Support organization that offers many free services.

Overeaters Anonymous
1-800-743-8703

For Further Reading

Eagles, Douglas A. *Your Weight.* New York: Franklin Watts, 1982.

Kane, Jane Kozak. *Coping with Diet Fads.* New York: Rosen Publishing Group, 1990.

Kubersky, Rachel. *Everything You Need to Know about Eating Disorders: Anorexia and Bulimia.* New York: Rosen Publishing Group, 1992.

Lukes, Bonnie L. *How to Be a Reasonably Thin Teenage Girl.* New York: Atheneum, 1986.

McFarland, Rhoda. *Coping with Self-Esteem*, rev. ed. New York: Rosen Publishing Group, 1993.

Moe, Barbara. *Coping with Eating Disorders.* New York: Rosen Publishing Group, 1991.

Index

63

About the Author
Karen Bornemann Spies was an elementary school teacher and vice principal before embarking on a second career in publishing. She has written school curriculum as well as several books for young people. Ms. Spies teaches writing at the community college level and offers workshops for young writers. She lives with her husband and two children in Colorado.

Acknowledgments and Photo Credits
Cover photo by Chuck Peterson.
Photo on page 56: Jill Heisler Jacks; all other photos by Dru Nadler.
Chart on page 36 by Sonja Kalter.

Design/Production: Blackbirch Graphics, Inc.